Yoga, Path of Life

Yoga, Path of Life

Tashirat Teachers' Manual

Part I
Yoga, the Path of Life

Part II
Simply Simple Live Food Recipes

Artimia Arian

iUniverse, Inc.
New York Lincoln Shanghai

Yoga, Path of Life
Tashirat Teachers' Manual

iUniverse books may be ordered through booksellers or by contacting:

iUniverse
2021 Pine Lake Road, Suite 100
Lincoln, NE 68512
www.iuniverse.com
1-800-Authors (1-800-288-4677)

ISBN-13: 978-0-595-39862-1 (pbk)
ISBN-13: 978-0-595-84260-5 (ebk)
ISBN-10: 0-595-39862-6 (pbk)
ISBN-10: 0-595-84260-7 (ebk)

Printed in the United States of America

Part I
Yoga, the Path of Life

Dedication

I dedicate this book to all students willing to aspire to the highest—the Path of Life; to all those who have the dedication and discipline required to walk this greatest path.

Contents

Preface and Acknowledgements

I thank two great Yoga teachers, Swami Sivananda and Swami Vishnudevananda. I am immensely grateful for their love and instruction in Yoga, in Life.

Tashirat Cosmic Yoga Teachers' Training Basic Level and Level 1

INTRODUCTION

To teach, one has to live one's teaching; one has to vibrate the teaching so as to be an example of it. Preaching is not teaching. One's own example will inspire and teach others. Yoga teachers must therefore be Yoga practitioners.

We are all students forever; we must all strive to learn forever. Knowledge is infinite, thus no subject can ever be fully mastered. However once a certain level of mastery of any subject has been attained, it is our obligation to impart that knowledge to those who are receptive to it. Life is an interaction of give and take. Our cups need to be emptied in order to be replenished.

Yoga signifies union: the integration within the individual of the 3 vehicles (physical, emotional and mental bodies), the strengthening and balancing of these bodies; the integration and harmonious interaction of the individual with other individuals; and the highest union, the union of the individual spirit with the Universal Spirit.

Ideally Yoga teachers have dedicated their lives to God putting aside their own personal desires. "Thy will my Lord, not my will" characterizes the attitude of a true Yogi. However in order to live God's Will, one has to be connected to the Universal Spirit, and clearly hear God voice so as to be guided by It in one's own life and in one's guidance of others.

No books, no knowledge is Absolute. Times change, the essence of the book may be correct, but the knowledge must be applied and adapted to each unique individual and to each different epoch. This is only feasible if the teacher is connected, is guided in his/her work. The Yoga teacher must be ever aware that s/he is an instrument working for a Divine Cosmic Plan and as such all work is guided and surrendered to that Plan. Only in this manner is the work valuable on a Cosmic scale.

Hence the singular aim of a Yogi and a Yoga teacher, is to raise his/her vibration so as to achieve this connection with God or the Universal Spirit. This aim is achieved through the daily practice of ancient scientific Yoga techniques, in addition to the purification of one's diet and the scrupulous observance of ethics and morals.

Yoga, Union, represents Chakra 6. Chakra 6 is the positive cosmic pole which corresponds to Life. The Yoga teacher thus guides the student in all the chakra lessons (refer to Cosmic Reawakening by Artimia Arian), possessing a thorough knowledge of them, having mastered them him/herself Yoga is the Chakra 6 lesson. The mark of an outstanding Yoga teacher, is one who lives and vibrates all that Chakra 6 embodies. This is the challenge of all Yoga teachers.

Correct diet and physical exercise (which could include dynamic Yoga practice such as Ashtanga Yoga) is the basis of our Kundalini Human Energy. Diet and exercise relate to Chakra 3, the Solar Plexus, the human energy battery. Physical body nourishment is a sorely neglected area in general on Earth, attributing to the widescale chronic diseases. A Yoga teacher must possess this fundamental knowledge so as to impart it to all students. How can a Yoga teacher, a teacher of Life, be a flesh-eater or sugar consumer, or not guide his/her disoriented students, providing them with logical information and improved alternative habits? Ahimsa, non-violence is one of the most highly respected principles in Yoga. Truncating the evolutionary path of animals for the appeasement of one's own tastebuds is not recommended. Every positive act of creation augments one's force; every destructive act diminishes it.

Teaching Techniques

INTRODUCTION

Before embarking upon the myriad details which comprise a good Yoga class, let it be remembered that the tone of the class, set by the teachers vibration, is of prime importance. The vast majority of students in an open class are ignorant as to many of the finer details of the postures or pranayama, but all students FEEL the class atmosphere. All Yoga teachers should practice 15–20 minutes of pranayama, in preparation, before teaching a class.

In Tashirat we recommend Level I for beginners and for open classes. The Level I consists of the Sivananda 12 basic postures, although the headstand is reserved for more intermediate students. The open class consists of Kapalabhati, Anuloma Viloma (both Pranayama exercises), followed by the classical Sun Salutation, a minimum of 9 or 10 of the 12 basic postures and some variations thereof concluding with a final relaxation.

Level 1 is a slow, meditative practice, attuning the student to the physical body and increasing concentration. As most beginners have little body consciousness, and as most people are inclined to be distracted by the senses the eyes are closed in Level I, withdrawing the senses and heightening concentration, extinguishing the left brain. In the Level 1 practice it is the right brain, the intuitive mind that is brought to the fore. The Cosmic feminine passive energy of let go, surrender is emphasized.

We do not advise beginners to initiate their Yoga practice with a dynamic more Kundalini Energy type practice, as there is a strong probability of unnecessary injury. One requires bodily awareness, correct breathing and the adept use of the breath in the postures as a basic pre-requisite, before advancing to a dynamic practice. In Level I one learns how to work the "let go" energy in one's practice and in one's life. The student is guided never to push himself to the limit of pain. S/he slowly and cautiously edges forward to a comfortable position and then by working the breath, in particular the relaxation with each exhalation, the posture is improved and the student is able to find his/her limit in the position, without experiencing pain.

The energy which still predominates on Earth today is the masculine, human Kundalini Energy which is characterized by dynamic activity and force to achieve success. The Earth, however, has shifted into a higher vibration, one which corresponds to Chakra 4, and is therefore closer in proximity to the Chakra 6 feminine Cosmic Energy than to Chakra I, the masculine Kundalini Energy. As our programming for generations has been precisely this masculine human outward tendency, we initiate our practice in Tashirat with the opposite energy, the energy of surrender, the inward focus, the Cosmic Energy, to counteract the imbalance present globally on Earth, and evident in most individuals.

We have commenced the Transition Years (approximately 2000–2010). The closer we move to the year 2010, the less Human World (Kundalini Energy) programming will be effective, and the more Cosmic World (Cosmic Energy) programming will yield success. Through the years Mother Earth will be moving up towards Chakra 6. The more in tune one is with Her vibration, the more rewarding these Transition Years. The energy to be fostered in these years is the meditative, unstressful, harmonious, loving, feeling Cosmic Energy. This is the energy which is elicited in the Level I Tashirat Yoga class. The class is patterned on the Sivananda teaching, the class structure and sequence being ideal for beginners.

The Yoga Salon

The arrangement of one's teaching space is of primary importance. The room must be well ventilated and spacious. Ideally all Yoga mats and students face the same direction, this being advantageous to the energy flow. The room should be painted in white or light elevating colors and free of disturbing accessories. Live plants, flowers and well selected paintings are suitable adornments.

To set the tone of the class, appropriate music is played and incense is lit. The teacher arrives 15–20 minutes before the class, to check the order and cleanliness of the salon, to arrange the yoga mats and to do his/her pranayama. As students arrive, greet them with a smile and indicate which mat they should use, but try and refrain from much talking. Avoid socialization before the class. Students can warm up or recline in savasana (the relaxation pose).

If the Yoga school provides the Yoga mats, it is best for the teacher to arrange them prior to the entrance of the students. Before commencing the class, endeavor to group the beginners, intermediate and advanced students, to facilitate teaching.

Start the class punctually, even if there are few students. Begin with three Oms and then a prayer in Sanskrit or the language of the country. The pranayama and prayer elevate and balance the teacher's vibration, the student's vibration and the environment.

The Class Structure

The teacher has the option of beginning the class with pranayama or of initiating with preliminary warm-up exercises such as eye and/or neck exercises, hip openers (e.g. butterfly), any forward bend and a sitting spinal twist. If they are not done before the pranayama they should be incorporated after pranayama, before the Sun Salutation.

The class structure for an Open Class is as follows:

> 5–10 mins. Warm-up exercises.
>
> 10–15 mins. Pranayama.
>
> 15 mins. Sun Salutation.
>
> 45 mins. Asanas.
>
> 10 mins. Final Relaxation and Meditation.

Follow the Sivananda sequence of asanas. In Level 1 the Dolphin is used as a preparation for the Headstand, The Fish must always follow the Shoulderstand and Plough. Forward Bend variations can be inserted before Paschimottanasana, the classical Forward Bend. The Cobra works the upper back. The Locust, the lower back. The Bow works the upper, middle and lower back. The closer the knees are in the Bow, the more the stretch is moved into the upper back, avoiding lower back compression. If back bend variations are incorporated, bear this information in mind and insert the variations in the correct places. The Spinal Twist follows, proceeded by the Crow or any other balancing posture. The Triangle or other lateral back muscle exercises ensue. Standing postures could be implemented at this point. Final Relaxation concludes the class.

How long does one hold the asanas ?

Technically an asana is a pose that is held for a minimum of one minute. However, it is always advisable to adapt the class to your students and not attempt to adapt students to rigid rules. Always advice students, beginners in particular, to come out of a pose if you observe they are over-exerting (trembling muscles, unrelaxed breathing).

The more advanced the students, the longer they will be able to hold the asanas comfortably. The longer one holds a pose, the more benefits one reaps. It is difficult to maintain a motionless posture, as the nature of the mind is unsteady. The mind loathes routine, discipline and lack of variety. It is difficult for the mind to hold the pose.

Meditative Hatha Yoga purifies and trains the abstract, intangible mind, by working the mind's concrete manifestation, the physical body. By stilling the body, by deepening the respiration, one calms and centers the mind. The mind must be one hundred percent present in every second of the Yoga class (the teacher's mind and the students' minds).

How long is the relaxation period between postures ?

This too depends on the students. The more advanced students have learnt how to relax in the asanas and therefore require less relaxation between postures. For beginners one observes their abdominal breathing. When their breath has returned to normal, the next asana is announced.

Sanskrit Prayers and Names

It is a good idea to use the Sanskrit asana names in a class for various reasons:

1. The Sanskrit alphabet consists of the 50 root sounds in the universe, and as such it is a language very close to telepathy. It is known as devangari, the language of the gods.

2. By repeating the asana's Sanskrit name in addition to the English or Spanish name, the students become familiar with the Sanskrit names, which are useful when giving a class to students of varying nationalities.

16

3. *Initiating the class with a Sanskrit prayer is very powerful and connects the teacher to his/her teachers and lineage.*

Kapalabhati

Kapalabhati is considered to be one of the six kriyas (purificatory exercises) and a variety of pranayama (breathing exercises). It is diaphragmatic breathing, especially used to control the movements of the diaphragm. It is therefore excellent for asthmatics who tend toward superficial thoracic respiration. It is a blood purifier, enabling large quantities of carbon dioxide to be eliminated and much fresh oxygen to be inhaled. The forceful pumpings stimulate the stomach, liver and pancreas.

Pranayama is always performed before the Sun Salutation and Asanas because in Kapalabhati the energies are awakened in the Solar Plexus and on each retention, are directed to the higher energy centers. In Anuloma Viloma the two energies, the masculine and the feminine energies, are balanced.

In Tashirat we teach Cosmic Kapalabhati, which differs from the Classical Kapalabhati only in the mudras and positioning of the hands.

TECHNIQUE

Sitting in a comfortable crossed-legged position, with the back straight, chest out, shoulders back and chin slightly tucked in, ensuring a perfect spine alignment, the students are instructed to close their eyes and attempt to keep them closed throughout as much of the class as possible. The hands are relaxed upon the knees, palms up. More advanced students are encouraged to practise the lotus or half lotus.

The teacher never closes his/her eyes during the class, permitting him/her to always be aware of and sensitive to all the students all the time, thus being able to guide and assist them.

Teacher: Inhale, abdomen inflates like a balloon (abdomen out), exhale, abdomen relaxes (abdomen in). Inhale a full deep breath, exhale. Inhale and begin.

The pumpings begin. At this point the students' hands are placed in the Unifying Mudra (Cosmic), directly in front of the Solar Plexus without touching the body, the thumbs are just below the sternum. In the Unifying Mudra, the fingertips of both hands are gently touching, fingers slightly curved and apart. The elbows are out, open, away from the body but relaxed (not rigid).

For the pumpings the teacher repeats "one" with a lot of prana for each exhalation. S/he must explain to any new students that s/he will be verbalizing the exhalations but that the students do not use the voice, only the breath, although the exhalations are strong and forceful. It is best to do a quick demonstration for beginners. Rhythm must increase towards the end of the round of pumps and voice must change so students know the round is coming to an end.

In Kapalabhati the emphasis is on the forceful short exhalations. The exhalations are active and are one quarter of the inhalations. The inhalations occur naturally, passively and silently, by releasing and relaxing the abdominal muscles immediately after the contractions.

The number and speed of the pumpings vary according to the students present. The more advanced the students, the more rapidly they are able to execute the contractions, and the more pumpings they will be able to perform. In a mixed intermediate open class, one could do 35 pumpings the first round, 50 the second and 70 the third. The breath is retained for one minute, or more for more advanced students (teacher use a watch with a second hand). However emphasize that one is never to force the breath. Whenever the student needs to exhale, s/he does so, inhaling and retaining again when able. Students must inhale and exhale twice before retaining.

During the contractions the focus is on the solar plexus and the hands in front of the solar plexus. During the first retention the prana and the hands are moved to Anahata Chakra (4th). During the second retention to Visudha Chakra (5th) and finally on the third retention to Ajna Chakra (6th).

TEACHING TIPS

1. *The most common error is that students fail to release and relax the abdominal muscles after contractions. They therefore create abdominal tension and are unable to do many pumpings.*

2. *Ensure that beginners are not hyperventilating i.e. inhaling sucking the abdomen in and exhaling and relaxing it.*

3. *Provide suitable cushions for students who are incapable of sitting cross-legged comfortably. If the knees are raised more than two fingers from the floor, provide a cushion, facilitating the opening of the hips.*

4. *Correct the sitting position by opening up the shoulders, straightening the back and centering the head. Only correct during the contractions, never whilst the student is retaining the breath.*

5. *If there are only one or two beginners in the class, do not waste the class' time with a class demonstration. Ask them to practise abdominal breathing until the rest of the students are retaining their breath. Then very quietly use the one minute retention time to demonstrate and explain to the beginners, or any other student who you observe to be committing errors.*

6. *The teacher's pumping indications ("one") must be rhythmical and not loud, but filled with prana. The teacher should be exhaling at the same time as the students, thereby generating a strong group energy. The rhythm of the pumpings can increase toward the end of each round and each round can also be slightly faster than the last.*

7. *Throughout the class give concise, clear instructions, enabling the students to easily follow the class with eyes closed. AVOID THE TENDENCY OF TALKING TOO MUCH.*

8. *Always bearing in mind that a large percentage of a Meditative Yoga class should be silent, some of the silent periods can be used to explain the benefits of the pranayama or the asana, or to enrich the students with other interesting related knowledge.*

9. *Moola Bandha can be taught to more advanced students only.*

Anuloma Viloma

Deep breathing is a great preventor of colds, flu, etc. Shallow breathing is linked to colds, sinus problems and unhealthy emotional state caused through nervous tension etc. Good ventilation is essential throughout a Yoga class. The windows may be closed during the final relaxation, as the body temperature drops.

Most people breathe incorrectly, inhaling raising the shoulders and pulling in the abdomen. Air is our primary food and medicine, more essential than solid food or water. Correct breathing is basic to mastering the art of happy, harmonious and productive living. In Level I we first teach abdominal breathing, as so few people naturally breathe properly. A complete Yogic breath consists of abdominal, thoracic and clavicular breathing. This corresponds to the Cosmic Breath, the true Breath of Life. Thus breathing in Level 1 is a continual focal point, always emphasized. Teachers, really work on perfecting your students' breathing habits, which must obviously be transferred to their lives.

ANULOMA VILOMA OR ALTERNATE NOSTRIL BREATHING

The breath naturally alternates between two nostrils. It alternates approximately every hour and fifty minutes in healthy people. Due to incorrect living habits, actually in most people this change of breath from one nostril to the other varies a great deal.

The breath in the right nostril is hot, according to the Yogis. The left nostril breath is cool. The right nadi is the sun breath or pingala, and the left nadi the moon breath or ida. The energy that flows through pingala nadi produces heat in the body, is catabolic and accelerates the body organs. Ida nadi is cooling, anabolic and inhibitory to the body organs. When the breath flows for more than two hours through one nostril, an imbalance of excess heat or cold will result in the body.

The main purpose of Anuloma Viloma is to balance the two energies found in the body and in the universe—the catabolic, male kundalini energy and the anabolic, female, cosmic energy.

TECHNIQUE

The Cosmic mudras will be used. The index fingertip of the right hand forms a circle by touching the fingertip of the right thumb. The knuckle of the right thumb is placed just below the nasal bone, gently closing off the right nostril. The left hand is positioned in front of Anahata Chakra, the thumb in front of the base of the sternum. A circle is formed with the thumb and index finger of the left hand too. The three remaining fingers of both hands are directed upwards, channeling the energy flow to the higher chakras. On the breath retention, the mudras remain, but the right hand is centered in front of Ajna Chakra. The elbows are extended outward, raising the energy flow, but they are light and relaxed. If the arms hurt, lower them, rest them and raise them again when comfortable.

One round consists of exhaling through the left nostril, inhaling left, retaining, exhaling right, inhaling right, retaining and exhaling left. At least 5 rounds should be completed in a Level I class. The ratio of inhale: retain: exhale is 1:4:2. So if you inhale to a count of 4, you would retain to a count of 16 and exhale to a count of 8. The exhalation is always double the inhalation. If you find the retention time is too difficult for beginners, alter the ratio a little, perhaps to 1: 3: 2. The exhalation is however always twice the length of the inhalation.

The focus is on Ajna Chakra (6th). The 5 rounds are followed by a minute of silence at least. Music is never utilized during Pranayama, but it can be used after the minute of silence. The students are instructed to either lie down or remain seated during the silent time, give them the option.

THE MUDRA SIGNIFICANCE

The index finger represents the individual ego. The illusory ego that makes one want to segregate oneself from the All; the ego that makes one focus on one's differences, one's superiority or inferiority in comparison to others; the *ego that wants to prove itself right always; the ego that fights only for itself and its own; the ego that always seeks recognition.*

The thumb represents the Universal Spirit. The individual ego thus unites to the Universal Spirit forming a circle, one of the basic units of life. A circle is force. It has no beginning and no end. Life is full of circles, representing the cycles we travel—cycles of activity and great action, abundance of Kundalini Energy; cycles of passivity, of nurturing oneself, reflection, meditation and learning, Cosmic Energy. A cycle has no clear beginning or end; the termination of one cycle merges slowly into the initiation of the next. The transition should always be smooth and gradual.

Think of all the circular things in Nature—the atom, the cell which is the basic structural living unit of life, the energy centers, the planets, the sun, the moon. If you throw a stone into a pond, it produces circular ripples. Circles, circular movements, are gentle, without any sharp, aggressive angles. Circles expand, they do not penetrate as do the pointed triangles, they expand. But circles too are composed of tinier circles, points, which comprise the line of the circle, the periphery.

In this Cosmic Era, the Earth has moved into Chakra 4, and continues to ascend. Our focus is on group work. Compare a group to a multicellular organism, as opposed to the individual, a unicellular organism. A multicellular organism is more effective as specialization occurs—different parts of the organism (group) are endowed with different talents, and perform different functions. It is more effective, more productive, due to the division of labor. Its chances of survival are greater, as if anything happens to one cell (one person), immediately others take on its labor.

A point, a singe individual, expands tremendously when s/he unites to other points, other individuals, with the same goals. In this way a circle is formed, a Circle of Force. A Circle of Force must be a circle of love, of sincerity, of openness, in which there is transparency.

All interactions and decisions are transparent. Everything is voted and the majority vote is respected. People communicate directly rather than to a third party, behind a person's back.

25

There is space within and without the circle for the members to breathe. The rules are the rules of love and life, beyond that each is a free, unique individual, entitled and encouraged to live life to the full in his/her very own way. Life must be lived, without anyone feeling restricted or pressurized by the circle. Only in this way will each individual flow, evolve, be happy and be able to contribute a great force to the circle. An individual's force is his/her love and happiness, his/her constant joy.

The circle can then be a Circle of Force as the individuals composing the circle are beings who are joyful, creative and each choosing to do what s/he wants to do, each loving his/her activity and therefore each always contributing to the circle with a force of love and joy. This makes for a strong, happy Circle of Force. A circle has no point denoting the head.

A Circle of Force must be comprised of members who are in Chakra 4 or above. If the members have gaping holes in any of the lower chakras, these will act as impediments for themselves and others, in their own evolution and in the evolution of the Circle. Thus as a Chakra 4 individual, each individual's aim will be to dedicate his/her life to God and God's Divine Plan. Each one's aim will be to ascend to Chakra 6, the highest level of entrega and discipline, in order to clearly receive and comprehend God's will and obey it. One's greatest and sole desire and joy will be one's service to humanity and one's own on-going evolution, capacitating one to enrich one's service infinitely.

In a true Circle of Force there is no head as such, there is a communal unity of affinity, friendship, sharing, a spirit of helping, a strongly cemented bond of love between all the members. This strong bond is created by no-one ever criticizing another (even in thought); by no-one ever listening to criticism of a circle member or anyone else; by nobody stepping out of line, attempting to be a dominant figure, minimizing the worth of other circle members; by no one member or select members making the decisions. The circle's strength is in its regularity, not irregularity. A circle, like a wheel, cannot ride smoothly if it is irregular, manifesting a point or points which are outstanding. Therefore let each circle member contribute freely and uninhibitedly with all sincerity, to the circle of love. Let the circle be such a force that the members' growth is never inhibited, only strengthened by the circle.

For a circle to be one of great force, each member has to be working on him/herself, on every level, transforming him/herself into a dynamic force.

Never resort to trivialities. Let love and real understanding be the circle's foundation.

A functioning Circle of Force enables the circle members to firstly accelerate their own growth and secondly help many others to do the same. It can only be achieved through love, sharing, giving, caring and above all laughter and happiness. No circle member is superior or inferior to any other in any way. The wheel of love (the circle) will then be able to ride smoothly through humanity and it will leave its firm track of love, life, happiness and light, wherever it goes. The underlying strength and the individual work of each circle member is what will determine the force of the circle. The bottom line is that each circle member must be consistently, continuously, doing his/her own spiritual practice, so that s/he can be a valuable individual force, contributing to the greater United Force of All.

Returning to the mudra in Analoma Viloma, a circle which symbolizes uniting yourself to others for the good of humanity and uniting yourself to God, is what is signified by the union of the index finger symbolizing the ego, with the thumb, symbolic of God. The other three fingers represent the three vehicles of man. The middle finger, the longest, characterizes the densest body, the physical. The ring finger is symbolic of the emotional body and the little finger the mental body. The three vehicles have to be strengthened and purified to such an extent that they can then be transcended, and the ultimate Union of the individual to the All can transpire. The bodies can be transcended when they are balanced, as they are no longer obstacles in the aspirant's evolution, and in the aspirant's connection with God.

The Sun Salutation

The movements must be well co-ordinated with the breath. The first two to four rounds can be done slowly as the body warms up, providing all the finer position details. The next four rounds can be unguided, provided there are no first-timers. The teacher is given the opportunity to correct the students individually. Suitable music should be played. One round consists of the twelve positions, if the right leg is moved back in position 4, the right leg is again moved forward in position 9. The next round the legs are alternated.

A few important details for each position:

Position 1—Perfect standing position, feet together, chest open, shoulders back, lower back arch but not too exaggerated i.e. tuck in the pelvis. Inhale, exhale hands in the Unifying Mudra.

Position 2—Open arms up and back, hands in Unifying Mudra. Contract buttocks to protect lower back as one arches the upper back. The backbend should work the upper back muscles, not compress and damage the lower back (a common beginner error that teachers must be on the look out for). Work the arms, moving them as far back as possible, without arching the lower back, for beginners. Even for more advanced students, the stretch is mostly in the upper and middle back. If the student does not have the flexibility in the arms, the hands can be separated but the arms should be straight. The head tilts back and the neck is relaxed. (Neck exercises must have been completed before the Sun Salutation).

Position 3—If the student wishes to work the ham strings then the legs would be straight even if s/he does not have the flexibility to touch the floor with the hands. With each exhalation the hands are inched a little lower. If the lower back is to be worked, bend the knees if necessary and press the palms into the floor. Slowly work on straightening the legs as much as possible. The chin is moved forward towards the feet, as in any forward bend; the chest moves towards the thighs and knees.

Position 4—Stretch the right leg back, ensuring that the left knee does not fall to the side, avoiding the stretch. The knee is in line with the ankle. Open the chest, shoulders back. The back foot can be flat or the toes can be tucked under. The hands can be placed palms flat down or up on the finger tips. Variations can be inserted at this point e.g. crescent moon, standing postures, splits, etc.

Position 5—Left leg back, body perfectly straight in a pushup position. Buttocks are neither raised, nor sagging. Head up.

Position 6—Drop the knees and chest to the floor, without moving them forward or backward. If the chest cannot touch the floor owing to lack of flexibility, then move the chest slightly forward. Elbows close to the body. Chin or forehead touches the floor. Lower back totally arched, buttocks raised high.

Position 7—Cobra. For beginners it is best to have them raise their hands a few cms off the ground in Cobra, protecting the lower back. The beginner tendency is to lift up into Cobra with straight arms, compressing the lower back. This must be avoided by aware teachers. The Cobra is an upper back stretch. One must feel the student's hard upper and middle back muscles to ensure this stretch. The lower back is relaxed. Maintaining the heels touching protects the lower back too. Most people possess a tight, closed upper back (the emotional area) and they tend to overcompensate by overworking the lower back, frequently injuring it. Teachers must be conscious of protecting the lower back throughout the class.

Position 8—Downward dog. Try to move the stretch into the upper back and shoulder region. Head can be up or down, according to the stretch desired. Try to work the heels down.

The Sun Salutation mantras can be repeated by the teacher, co-ordinating them with the movements, each movement terminating with Namah. The mantras can be found in the Sivananda Chant Book—Surya Namaskara.

The Sun Salutation should be accelerated with each round as it is a body warm-up exercise, preparing for the asanas. Ashtanga Sun Salutations can be used for more advanced students.

Teach beginners the classical Sun Salutation. Add a variation option only after the first few rounds of the classical Sun Salutation. Only give 1–2 variations to the Sun Salutaion otherwise it is difficult for students to remember the sequence on their own and they are too preoccupied to warm up.

Correct arms in Sun Salutation. Palms should be facing each other and arms should be straight.

Never stop a student during Sun Salutation and have him/her go back to something s/he did incorrectly. Wait for the next round and correct in the moment.

The Final Relaxation

The final relaxation is the climax of the class. 10–15 mins. is dedicated to it. Incense is lit, windows and doors are closed. Covering oneself, either with a blanket/sweater and socks to keep the body warm is suggested and appropriate music is essential.

The students are instructed to tense and relax every body part, commencing with the grosser parts, moving from the feet upward, towards the finer facial muscles. The students then mentally relax each body part e.g. Teacher: feel the energy moving into the knees and thighs, knees and thighs relax, mentally repeat the order three times, commanding the knees and thighs to relax.

This part is extremely important. Our automatic (involuntary) nervous system is divided into the sympathetic and parasympathetic nervous system. The sympathetic system prepares the body for the "fight or flight" response, pumping adrenalin, increasing the respiration and heartbeats, increasing the blood to the muscles, etc. The parasympathetic system relaxes, it is the counterbalance of the sympathetic. However most of us live in a continual state of "fight or flight" due to our stressful lifestyles. Traffic, the telephone or doorbell ring, negative thoughts, worry, etc. all trigger off the sympathetic nervous system. It is imperative that we consciously activate the parasympathetic nervous system, relaxing the organism that has been overextenuated and overstimulated. It is important that the student sends the commands to his/her own subconscious, and does not merely receive the instructions from the teacher.

The teacher then receives a visualization and/or a significant message to impart, the duration of which can be 3–5 minutes. The class must end in silence, no talking, no music. The student is given the opportunity to transcend the three bodies—the physical body having been worked, now relaxes; the student is feeling positive and happy after having accomplished a good class, the emotions are balanced; the mind can be peaceful and calm. The students are encouraged not to sleep: to relax deeply but remain conscious.

In Tashirat we end all classes with a 15–20 minute meditation which initiates or terminates with a short prayer or reading. Ideally the class should end with a meditation, the length depending on the time available.

Useful Teaching Tips

1. *It is very important that teachers are clean and well groomed. Teachers must shower before the class, clean and trim nails/toenails, wear very clean white clothes, and tie hair back neatly. It's a good idea to wear socks on the way to class so your feet stay clean.*

2. *Giving a bilingual class is an art. Do not tire the students by repeating everything in both languages. The class is mostly given in one language, the elected language depending on the language spoken by the majority. Instructions such as inhale and exhale are understood by all students in any language. Only the essential instructions are repeated in both languages. All qualified Tashirat teachers have to be able to give a bilingual class—in English and in the language of the country.*

3. *Giving an open class is not easy as it usually consists of a mixture of beginners, intermediates and advanced students. The real art lies in keeping each student working at his/her level, stimulated and comfortable i.e neither bored nor intimidated by postures that are too difficult. Beginners have little body consciousness and are therefore vulnerable to injuries as they attempt to do any posture and to hold postures too long, unless otherwise instructed by the teacher. Beginners are gently instructed to relax, whilst other students are given variation options or requested to hold postures. For example advanced students could be doing the headstand (holding for 5 minutes or doing variations) while the teacher guides other students in a headstand preparation such as the dolphin or in the 8 headstand steps. The key is to be focusing on the student you're working with but always keep an eye on all the other students. Never spend too long on one student. All students want and require attention, regardless of their level. Advanced students must be introduced to new variations, and their asanas must be corrected in detail. Although many students may be working on different variations of an asana, all students are kept on the same asana.*

4. *Asana correction. Students learn more by feeling a correction than by lengthy explanations. Students must all be constantly corrected in their postures, this is what they come to class for. Teachers give instructions and then walk around correcting postures. Do not give more attention to beginners. Give equal attention to all students. It is a good idea to place a beginner next to or behind an intermediate student and tell him to follow him. When a class consists of more than 20 students it is difficult to correct all students. The teacher must be very clear with the verbal instruction so that they are understood by all. When correcting a posture, ask the student to inhale and then exhale, adjusting them always on the exhale, as the student relaxes the muscles.*

5. *A quick teacher demonstration is sometimes necessary, avoiding long-winded explanations. Do not demonstrate if the students know the postures. Teachers never do their asanas in class. Do not use the class as your practice period or to exhibit your asana ability, it could intimidate beginners. Only demonstrate when appropriate and necessary.*

6. *Give proper specific instructions. E.g. if you are having the class do down dog, and lift a leg, you must specify if you want them to open the hips or keep hips squared etc. You must know what you are working and guide the class accordingly.*

7. *Do not interrupt a class by giving specific instructions to a single student. Always walk up to the student and talk in a low voice without disturbing others. Never lose awareness of the rest of the class when you are correcting a student. Never talk to a student while others are waiting for instruction.*

8. *Talking in excess is one of the commonest errors of most teachers. Yoga represents Chakra 6, silence, union, peace, harmony. Simple, essential, concise instructions, nothing more.*

9. *The teacher must be aware of everything throughout the class e.g. which foot must be brought forward in the sun salutation; how many pumpings you did in the first round of kapalabhati; how many rounds of analoma viloma you have done, etc.*

10. *Do not relax too long between postures, particularly in the morning, as the body cools down. 2–3 breaths should be sufficient, except for real beginners.*

11. *Be aware of the time throughout the class, abiding by the given class structure. Teachers must be punctual, beginning and ending classes on time always. The class must have an even flow, never rushing to fit in postures at the end of the class etc.*

12. *The voice intonations and volume are important. Do not talk too loud, it is tiresome and unrelaxing for students. Do not talk too softly, as students have to strain to hear and this too generates tension. Do not "sing" instructions. The volume and tone of the voice are directly related to ones vibration. A loud voice pertains to a teacher with an excess of Kundalini Energy and lack of Cosmic Energy. A Yoga teacher must possess a Chakra 5 vibration at least, without too many weaknesses in lower chakras, lowering the vibration. To achieve this the teacher must be working the Chakra 1–5 chakra lessons, whichever are pertinent to his/her life, in addition to purifying the diet and daily pranayama, asana and meditation practice. Selfless service is key to strengthening Chakra 4.*

13. *Music is a great tool if well used in Level I. It raises the class vibration and aids in relaxing and connecting students. The same music rehashed must be avoided. If utilized, the music must be well selected e.g. for sun salutation it could be dynamic, for final relaxation it cannot. The teacher must have different casettes prepared for different periods in the class. Music must not be played throughout the entire class, it can become disturbing. It must be used with great sensitivity, enhancing the class. Silence must be used too. It is also relaxing and elevating. Change the music for the final relaxation, announcing the transition.*

14. *Be sensitive to all students at all times e.g. do not leave students holding a posture too long whilst occupied in posture corrections.*

15. *When inserting variations, adhere to the Sivananda posture sequence. Ensure at least 9 of the 12 Sivananda basic postures. Always include some standing and balancing poses.*

16. *Always teach beginners how to somersault out of the headstand (assisted) before teaching the actual headstand. This helps the students to rid themselves of the fear of falling while in the headstand and teaches them how to fall correctly so they don't hurt themselves. Only teach the Dolphin to students who obviously don't have the upper body strength needed for the headstand.*

17. *Always inhale legs up and exhale legs down when doing legs lifts. Make sure students keep feet flexed and lower back is pressed down.*

18. *A good Yoga teacher-practitioner loves Yoga with a passion, and transmits that love to the students. An outstanding Yoga teacher is one who values Yoga, the union of the material and spiritual, above all else, and channels all his/her energies in this direction. His/her entire life is a manifestation of Yoga. A genuine Yoga teacher has initiated his/her journey on the Path of Life, the Path of Yoga, and is therefore capable of guiding the students on this highest of paths.*

"When the carnivorous diet is included in the human diet, the superior nature of people is obstructed, blunted and benumbed, and the internal flame of the spirit cannot give its light. This is a drastic rule for those who aspire to initiation and cannot be violated. When the student reaches a certain state in the spiritual path, it becomes necessary to discontinue in his diet all kinds of flesh foods and to put in a natural diet of fruit, fresh vegetables, greens, seeds and grains." (Ann Wigmore, *Naturama*, p.106)

Yoga is a most precise science and an art. It teaches the Art of Living. Tashirat signifies Truth, Love and Life. May all Tashirat teachers transform themselves into shining beacons of Truth, Love and Life, inspiring others to do the same.

Tashirat

Tashirat, the Path of Light,

Heralds only Truth in all its simplicity and clarity;

Lauds Love as the greatest constructive Force of Creation,

And Life as the ascending Evolutionary Spiral achieved by every positive

Thought, Word and Deed.

Tashirat, a Lighthouse of Knowledge,

A map to guide a wandering traveler back home

To a Land of Light,

A Land of Truth, Love and Life.

Artimia Arian

Part II

Simply Simple Recipes

Dedication

This book is dedicated to Gaia, Mother Earth, and all Her children who have the consciousness and dedication to recuperate and maintain vibrant, flexible, youthful bodies which are capable of housing an expanded consciousness. This book is dedicated to the dawn of a New Era of LIFE!

Contents

Preface and Acknowledgements

Very little on this book is original. Most credit goes to Ann Wigmore, one of the first live foods pioneers. I am ever indebted to her for all her research and the original, innovative, creative recipes she concocted. Most of these recipes are variations of her recipes.

Huge thanks to all my enthusiastic students and friends who have made raw food a part of their lives, and have shared ideas and recipes.

As live food is practically unheard of in Mexico, and books are unavailable, a practicle recipe book for the novice became necessity, facilitating the transition to live food eating in Mexico.

Amounts and measures have been deliberately omitted in most recipes, encouraging creativity and flexibility, according to personal tastes.

Required Live Food Kitchen Equipment

- Blender
- Dehydrator or Sun
- Juice Extractor
- Food Processor
- Chopping board and good knives
- Trays for sprouting and for bread making
- Cloths to cover the sprouts
- 2 large strainers—1 with a fine mesh for seed cheeses and for sprouting small seeds such as alfalfa; and 1 with a larger mesh for sprouting larger seeds such as wheat.

Note

1. ## To Disinfect

   i. For every liter of water add the juice of 2 lemons and 1 tbs. of sea salt. Wash the vegetables well and soak them in this water for 15 minutes.

   Or:

   ii. Place a small bundle of wheatgrass tied with a string or rubber band, in your soaking water. Wash the vegetables and soak them for 10–15 minutes.

2. ## To Sprout

   i.   Soak the seeds in a bowl of water overnight.

   ii. Remove the water in the morning using a large strainer.

   iii. Place the seeds in a large plate or tray and cover them with a humid cloth.

   iv. Wet the seeds and cloth twice a day, morning and night, never keeping them too wet, but never allowing them to dry.

   v.   Within 3–7 days (depending on the seeds) your sprouts will be ready. They are ready to eat once the first two green leaves appear.

   vi. They are best eaten fresh, but can be refrigerated in Tuppers or plastic bags.

3. *Condiments*

Bragg can be substituted with kelp, dulse (or any seaweed), tamari, soy sauce (diluted with warm water), miso, vegetable salt substitutes or sea salt. Refer to my book Cosmic Reawakening, the chapter "Useful Kitchen Tips and Simple Recipes" (pp. 117–118). In this chapter healthy substitutes and condiments are discussed in detail.

Salad Dressings

1. *Mexican Sauces*

   a) Blend:
      Guajillo chili
      Tomatoes
      Bragg
      Garlic and onion (optional)

   b) Blend:
      Green tomatoes
      Garlic
      Onion
      Cilantro
      Serrano Chili
      Bragg

   c) Blend:
      Tomatoes
      Onion
      Cilantro
      Bragg

      Dice:
      Tomatoes
      Onion
      Cilantro

      Mix everything together.

2. _Avocado Dressings (for approximately 1 lt. of dressing)_

   a) Blend:
       4 avocados
       Cilantro
       1 garlic clove
       Onion
       Juice of 2 lemons
       Fresh chili
       Water

   b) Blend:
       Avocado
       Basil
       Garlic
       Lemon
       Bragg
       Water

   c) Blend:
       Tahini
       Avocado
       Bragg
       Mint
       Water

3. _Carrot Tomato Dressing (for 1 lt.)_

Blend:
Olive oil
Water
Bragg
¼ large onion
1 tomato 1 large carrot
Small chili Serrano
Juice of 1 lemon
Little pure apple cider vinegar

4. *Light Sesame Seed Dressing*

   Blend:
   Sesame seed oil (or olive oil)
   Water
   Lemon
   Bragg
   Sesame seeds (sprouted)

5. *Garbanzo Dressing*

   Blend or homogenize in a food processor:
   Garbanzos (sprouted)
   Parsley
   Chives
   Garlic
   Celery
   Olive Oil
   Bragg
   Little water
   Bell Peppers

6. *Almond (or any other nut) Dressing*

   As above, substituting soaked nuts.

7. *Think, Creamy, Sunflower and/or Sesame Seed Dressing*

   Blend:
   Sprouted seeds (sunflower and/or sesame)
   Bragg
   Water
   Lemon
   Chili (optional)
   Herbs of choice

8. *Vegetable Dressing*

Blend vegetables of choice such as:
Tomatoes
Celery
Zucchini
Carrots
Cucumber
Bell Pepper
Herbs of choice
Oil
Bragg
Water
Lemon juice or pure vinegar (optional)
Garlic and/or onion

9. *Mayonnaise*

Blend:
½ cup lemon juice
2 tbs. Honey
2 tbs. Tahini
1/4 cup olive oil (or less)

10. *Spicy Dressing*

Blend:
Olive oil
Bragg
Water
Lemon juice
Fresh green chili
Cilantro

11. *Herb Dressing*

Blend:
Water

Bragg
Cilantro
Cayenne or fresh chili
Ginger powder and onion powder
Cumin
Italian herbs

Salads

1. *Salad:*
Mung and lentil sprouts, zucchini flower, watercress, cilantro, tomatoes, green pepper.

Dressing: Garbanzo or Nut dressing

2. *Coleslaw Salad:*
Shred any of the following and combine: cabbage, carrot, beet, radish, jicama, celery, red and green pepper.

Dressing: Mayonnaise or Avocado dressing

3. *Salad:*
Diced tomatoes, onions, chili Serrano, cucumbers.

Dressing: Oil, Bragg, garlic, lemon.

4. *Salad:*
Diced tomatoes, green peppers, onions, green beans, snow peas, celery, cauliflower, cilantro.

Dressing: Mexican Sauce c). Serve in large lettuce leaves with avocado and alfalfa sprouts.

5. *Green salad:*

- Lots of greens such as: watercress, large lettuce leaves, spinach leaves, finely chopped kale, arugula.

- Sprouts such as: radish, mung, lentil, trebol, and alfalfa.

- Add sliced tomatoes, grated carrots or jicama and any other vegetables such as radish cauliflower, mushrooms, etc.

Dressing: Avocado, sunflower seed or light sesame seed (or any of your choice).

6. *Salad:*
Finely chopped radish, fresh oregano, onion, cilantro, tomato.

Dressing: Bragg, lemon, olive oil, water.

7. *Salad:*
Large cubed tomato, jicama, bell peppers, celery. Add finely chopped Serrano chili.

Dressing: Garbanzo

8. *Salad:*
Mushrooms, onions, tomatoes, green peppers, cucumbers, jicama.

Dressing: Carrot Tomato Dressing

9. *Salad:*
Shredded spinach leaves topped with diced cucumber and tomato.

Dressing: Light Sesame Seed Dressing

10. *Salad:*
Diced kale, spinach, cilantro, parsley, watercress, tomatoes, onions, radishes.

Dressing: Tomatoes, Serrano chili, Bragg, oil.

11. *Stir Fry:*
    Cabbage, shredded
    Broccoli, chopped
    Carrots, julienne
    Celery, long, thin strips
    Red and Green bell peppers, finely sliced
    Mushrooms, finely sliced
    Ginger, finely sliced (small pieces)

    Dressing: Vinegar, Bragg, oil, orange juice.

Entrées

(To be combined with green salads)

1. Guacamole

2. Nopales

3. Ceviche

4. Taboule

5. Garbanzo Dip (or other seed dips)

6. Hamburger Patties

7. Spaghetti and Tomato Sauce

8. Gazpacho

9. Essene Bread Sandwiches

10. Seed Cheeses

11. Nut and Seed Loaves

12. Vegetable Loaves with Grains

13. Mock Tuna

14. Stuffed Vegetables

15. Tacos

Gaucamole

1. Dice: Tomatoes, onions, cilantro.

2. Mash avocados and add: Bragg, olive oil, lemon.

3. Mix everything together.

4. Variation: Add diced bell pepper (red and/or green), and celery.

Nopales

1. Soak small, tender nopales in warm water for a few hours until soft.

2. Dice and mix together: Nopales, tomatoes, onion, cilantro, radishes (optional).

3. Add: Olive oil and Bragg or sea salt.

Hot Mexican Nopales

1. Soak small, tender nopales in warm water.

2. Blend: Ancho chili, guajillo chili (seeds removed and soaked in warm water), garlic, onion, clove, oregano.

3. Cut nopales and mix with sauce and diced cilantro.

Ceviche

1. Dice and mix together: Mushrooms, tomatoes, onion, cilantro, fresh green chili.

2. Dressing: Bragg, lemon, olive oil.

3. Before eating break up small pieces of Nori sheets and add to the ceviche.

4. Variation: Add diced radish and red and/or green bell pepper.

Taboule

1. Dice and mix together: Tomatoes, onion or chives, green bell pepper, cucumber, watercress, parsley, mint, (or cilantro), olives, (optional).

2. Add: Sprouted wheat.

3. Dressing: Bragg, lemon, olive oil.

Garbanzo Dip

1. Homogenized in the food processor:

   Sprouted garbanzos (or any sprouted nuts or seeds), extra virgin olive oil, Bragg, lemon, garlic (optional), parsley and/or cilantro.

2. Add water for a creamier dressing, no water or very little for a thicker dip.

3. Variation: Add fresh chili for a spicy dip.

4. Variation: Add finely diced vegetables and herbs to the dip, e.g. diced onion, chives, carrots, celery, radish, bell peppers, cilantro or parsley.

5. Variation: Try adding other vegetables such as carrots, red peppers, chives, etc., when homogenizing in the food processor.

6. The dip can be used to stuff bell peppers or tomatoes or as a dip for broccoli and cauliflower flowerets and vegetable sticks such as carrots, celery, jicama, cucumber.

7. Variation: Add sprouted sesame seeds to the dip.

   Note: Garbanzos must be soaked for two nights in order for them to sprout. The water must be changed daily.

Hamburger Patties

1. Blend and sun dry in the form of patties:

    Sprouted lentils, sprouted wheat, Bragg, a variety of shredded vegetables such as carrots, beetroot, green pepper, celery, fresh chili, onion, garlic.

2. Add herbs and spices of choice, e.g. parsley, garlic, cilantro, basil, oregano, etc.

    Note: The patties can be dried to a hamburger.

3. Variation: Sprouted nuts and seeds can also be used instead of or together with the sprouted grains.

4. Patties can be sprinkled with sesame seeds or sunflower seed meal or almond meal, etc.

Spaghetti and Tomato Sauce

1. Dice: Red and green bell peppers, tomato, onion, fresh chili.

2. Add: Olive oil, kelp, tamari, fresh oregano and basil or dried Italian herb mix.

3. For tomato sauce, blend: Tomatoes, ½ avocado, onion, chili, tamari, oil.

4. Combine diced vegetables with the tomato sauce and serve over alfalfa sprouts or over spaghetti squash or zucchini finely shredded.

Gazpacho

Blend any of the following with or without water, depending on the desired consistency. If you wish to blend without water, start by blending the tomatoes, then add the rest.

1. Blend: Ripe tomatoes (many), cucumber, celery, red and green bell pepper, onion, garlic, fresh chili (optional), parsley, basil.

2. Can add olive oil and Bragg.

Combine well with an Essene bread sandwich.

Essene Bread Sandwiches

Essene Bread Preparation

1. Blend: Sprouted wheat, water, Bragg, cumin seeds, garlic, onion, guajillo chili, ancho chili (the seeds must be removed from the chilis and they must be soaked for a few hours before using).

2. Blend: ½ kg. Sprouted grain, 1 guajillo chili, 1 ancho chili, 2 tomatoes, Bragg or sea salt, chives, cumin seeds (few), 1 clove of garlic, oregano.

Sandwich Ideas

Top the bread with any of the following:

Guacamole
Garbanzo dip
Seed cheese
Avocado

Decorate the sandwiches with onion rings, radishes, tomato and bell pepper slices, alfalfa or trebol.

Seed cheeses

1. Blend equal amounts of sprouted sunflower seeds, sesame seeds and water. Allow the mixture to ferment for about eight hours at room temperature.

2. Place the mixture in a large strainer to drain for 1 to 3 days.

3. Finely chopped vegetables can be added to the seed cheese before or after fermentation. Good vegetables and herbs to use are: radishes, bell peppers (red and green), olives, garlic leaves (finely chopped), celery, parsley, cilantro, arugula.

4. Add kelp, Bragg, dried herbs or seaweed.

Nut and Seed Loaves

These are made in the same way as the seed cheeses. The nuts must be soaked overnight and peeled if possible (as in the case of almonds). The seeds are best soaked and sprouted.

1. The nuts-seed mixture can be left at room temperature to ferment, or eaten unfermented.

2. A wide variety of diced herbs and vegetables can be added to the seed loaves before or after fermentation.

3. The loaf can be placed in the sun or dehydrator for several hours if desired.

A Recipe Example:

1 ½ cups walnuts
1 ½ cups sunflower seeds
1 ½ cups almonds
1 tbs. minced garlic
½ tbs. sea salt
½ cup parsley, chopped
½ cup celery, chopped
1 tbs. onion, chopped
½ minced ginger (optional)
A little of any or all the following herbs:
Rosemary, tarragon, marjoram, minced
1 cup red bell pepper, chopped
1 tbs. (or less) jalapeño or Serrano chili

1 ½ tbs. (or less) cumin seeds
¼ cup olive oil

1. Blend the nuts and seeds with as little water as possible. Stir in the remaining ingredients.

2. Dehydrate or sun dry the loaf partially.

Good vegetables to use for nut-seed and grain loaves: red and green bell peppers, celery, mushrooms, red or white onions, garlic, carrots, beetroot, radishes.

Good herbs are: oregano, basil, parsley, cilantro, marjoram, rosemary, thyme.

Good sprouts for the loaves are: mung, lentil, garbanzo, sunflower, sesame, oats, wheat, barley, (or any other grain).

Vegetable Loaves with Grains

These are not fermented, but fermented seed cheese can be added for flavor.

1. Blend sprouted grains and add diced vegetable, e.g. sprouted oats blended with a little water.

2. Add grated carrots and diced green pepper, celery and onion. Mix with kelp, oregano and some seed cheese.

Mock Tuna

1. Homogenize in food processor:

    ½ cup sprouted oats (approximate measures to give idea of ratio of ingredients)
    ½ cup soaked almonds
    ½ cup sprouted sunflower seed (or seed cheese)
    Bragg, lemon, olive oil.

2. Dice about 3 cups (or more) of the following vegetables: Celery, red and green bell pepper, cilantro, fresh chili, chives, garlic.

3. Mix everything together or serve on large lettuce leaves (can be rolled in lettuce leaves and with sliced tomatoes.

Stuffed Vegetables

Vegetables such as bell peppers, tomatoes and avocados can be stuffed with:

1. Garbanzo or seed dips.
   Variation: mix dips with diced vegetables.

2. Guacamole.

3. Vegetable loaves.

4. Taboule.

5. Ceviche.

6. Sprouts or grated vegetables and dressings.

Tacos

Tacos can be created with large lettuce or spinach leaves or Nori sheets (seaweed) and a variety of fillings:

- Seed cheeses.

- Seed loaves.

- Garbanzo dips.

- Any grated vegetables or sprouts with a good dressing.

Soups

1. Blend: Green leaves (celery leaves, parsley, spinach, cilantro, arugula, kale, watercress, etc.), at least 1 cup of sprouts, fermented sunflower and sesame seeds, tomatoes, radish, chili (fresh), condiments.

2. Blend: 5 tomatoes, arugula, celery stems and leaves, parsley, chives, garlic, avocado, cauliflower. Add tamari or kelp and oil.

3. Blend: Tomato, cucumber, beet (a little), onion, cabbage leaves, spinach, dry vegetable seasonings, kelp or dulse.

4. Blend: Tomatoes, onion, red and green pepper, parsley, zucchini, celery, and vegetable seasoning. Add lentil sprouts to the blended soup.

5. Mix miso with water and add: sliced mushrooms, chives, and nori pieces.

6. Cut in the food processor to desired texture: broccoli, zucchini, cauliflower, carrots, celery, cabbage (and any other vegetables).

    Blend: Tomatoes, avocado, onion and garlic, Bragg, water.

    Dice: Cilantro, thyme, marjoram.

    Combine all ingredients.

7. For about 1 liter of soup blend: 2–4 tbs. olive oil, 1 cup water, Bragg, 10 small (or 5 large) carrots, 5 small tomatoes, 1 small lemon (the juice of).

Soups can be eaten at room temperature or warmed in the sun, ideal; heated very slightly on a low flame; or places in a Pyrex dish and then in a large bowl of hot water.

Sweets, Biscuits, Cake, Ice-Cream, Milk Drinks

Sweets

Candies and cookies can be created from ground or chopped dates, raisins, figs, nuts or seeds. Combine any soaked dried fruits with fresh fruits and nuts or seeds. Add powdered carob if desired. E.g. tahini and honey balls rolled in sesame seed. Refrigerate.

Biscuits (Cookies)

An endless variety of sweet cookies can be created in the same way as the Essene bread, e.g.

1. Blend: Sprouted wheat, carob powder, a little honey, walnuts, and banana.

2. Blend: Sprouted wheat (or any other grain), mango and banana, and cinnamon.

3. Blend: Sprouted wheat and raisins.

4. Blend: Sprouted wheat, coconut, pineapple, strawberries, and a little honey.

5. Combine: Tahini, honey, vanilla, wheat germ. Top with sesame seeds.

Cakes

Make the base (piecrust) from soaked flaxseeds and a little water. Top with a layer of tahini and honey. Top with any fresh or soaked dried fruit or fruit purées, e.g. apple purée and strawberry slices.

77

Different pies can be made from a crust of ground coconut or seeds and honey. Soaked dried fruit can be used as a binder. Any blended fruit sauce and/or chopped fruit can be used as a filling. Pies and cakes can be topped with rounds of bananas, kiwi, strawberries, etc., or berries (or nuts and seeds, raisins, etc.).

Blend soaked amaranth and oats, and mix it with tahini and honey. It can be cake or small cookies or smaller sweet balls. Sprinkle with sesame seeds and refrigerate.

In a large bowl mix: carrot pulp, raisins, walnuts, 1 day old sunflower seed sprouts (any other seeds or nuts), cinnamon, carob (optional, for a chocolate flavor). Add blended dates and carrot juice. Icing: orange juice, a little lemon juice, raw cashew nuts (unsalted)—blend.

Chi'ara's Apple Strudel

3 or 4 apples, peeled and finely chopped
2 orange peels, grated
1 lime
vanilla
cinnamon
1/3 cup raisins
1/3 kg. walnuts
1 cup dates

Blend walnuts and dates in food processor (or blender). This forms a base. Mix remaining ingredients in a bowl, adding more walnuts to flavor, if necessary. This is the strudel filling

Chi'ara's Carrot Cake

Blend: 2 cups pitted soaked dates, 2 cups tender coconut meat, ¼ cup ginger, enough carrot juice to blend it.

Add: 2 cups carrot pulp, 2 cups chopped walnuts, ½ cup raisins, cinnamon.

Crust base: Blend soaked almond and dates or prunes.

Icing: Blend ¼ kg. cashews, orange juice, a little honey.

Ice Cream

All ice-cream is made from peeled frozen fruit such as bananas, strawberries, cantaloupes, or any other fruit. Once frozen put it through a juicer or blender. Use a little water if using a blender or food processor. Different fruits can be mixed. Dates or raisins, cinnamon or carob can be added. Also try adding walnuts, almonds or sunflower seeds.

E.g. 2 frozen bananas, 3 dates, handful of walnuts—all blended.

Try blending banana and strawberry or banana and mango.

Milk Drinks

All milk drinks are made from sprouted nuts and/or seeds such as sunflower and sesame seeds or almonds. Blend the nuts and seeds in water. Add a little honey (or fruit such as banana and/or dates). Can be strained for milk or eaten unstrained as a thick milkshake mix. Cinnamon or carob can be sprinkled on top.

Breakfast Ideas

1. *Citric Fruit or Fruit Drinks,*
   any of which can be combined with 1–2 day sprouted sunflower or sesame seeds, or almonds soaked overnight and peeled.

   a) Sliced citric fruit with or without honey, e.g. oranges, pineapple, mandarin, grapefruit, and guava.

   b) Citric fruit salad with or without honey, combining 2–3 citric fruits, e.g. strawberry, kiwi, guava, pineapple, blueberries, etc. Can top it with whole or coarsely ground sprouted or soaked nuts or seeds.

   c) Blend citric fruit drinks combining 2–3 citric fruits, e.g. orange and pineapple; orange pineapple, and strawberry; orange and guava; strawberry and orange and/or mandarin juice diluted 50-50 with water.

2. *Melons,*
   watermelon, cantaloupe, sweet green melon.

3. *Breakfast Cereals,*

   a) Sprouted wheat, any sub-acid or sweet fruit (e.g. grated apple or sliced banana), any soaked dried fruit (e.g. dates, raisins, prunes), topped with honey and cinnamon or carob.

   b) Sprouted wheat blended with warm water and any sub-acid or sweet fruit, e.g. banana, apple, raisins, dates, figs, prunes. It can be strained if desired.

c) Sprouted wheat with soaked dried fruit of choice, topped with nut or seed milk. To make the nut or seed milk, blend the sprouted nuts or seeds with water. Strain if desired.

Add honey if desired.

4. *Nut-Seed Milks*

Juices

Raw vegetable juices are an essential supplement to a raw food diet (or any purification diet), particularly in the initial stages of the elimination of accumulated waste and the replenishment of the malnourished organism. All the nutritional elements and nutritional enzymes needed by the cells are found in the juices extracted from fresh raw vegetables, herbs, weeds, and fruits. The juices quickly furnish the body with all the necessary vitamins and minerals, minimal energy is utilized and they aid in regulating and normalizing the bowel movement.

Solid food requires many hours of digestion before its nourishment is available to the cells of the body, whereas in the form of juices, nutrients can be digested and assimilated in 10 to 15 minutes after ingestion, with minimum exertion of the digestive system. These juices are then almost totally employed in the nourishment and regeneration of the body's cells, tissues, glands and organs.

Fruit juices are the body cleansers, and they contain all the carbohydrate and sugar that the body requires. Vegetable juices are the body builders, containing all the amino acids, minerals, salts, enzymes and vitamins required by the body.

One can safely drink as much juice as one can comfortably drink without forcing oneself.

Good juice examples:

- ½ carrot, ½ spinach

- ½ carrot, ½ any other greens such as kale, watercress, parsley, celery stems and leaves. Beetroot leaves, green sprouts such as sunflower sprout greens. Use less of the strong greens such as parsley and watercress.

- ½ carrot, little beet, the rest celery.

- ¾ carrot (or less), ¼ cabbage (or more).

- ¾ carrot, ⅓ beet, ⅓ cucumber.

- V8 with a lot of tomatoes combined with any other vegetables such as celery, cucumber, parsley, bell pepper, sunflower greens, spinach, arugula. Can add lemon juice and a little Bragg or kelp to taste.

Daily Menu

Upon arising:
2–5 lemons in a glass (or less) of water.

Breakfast:
See breakfast Ideas.

Throughout the Morning: (10-11 am)
Any fruit.

Mid-Morning:
1–2 Vegetable Juices.

Lunch:
Salad and Dressing, Soup, or Entrée (refer to recipes).

Mid-Afternoon: (3-4pm)
1–2 Vegetable Juices.

Dinner: (6-7 pm)
As for Lunch or fruit.

Night:
Fruit.

Simple Food Combining Rules

1. *Fruit*

Acid and sour fruits (with the exception of lemon) should not be mixed with sweet fruits. Sub-acid fruits combine fairly well with either of these categories. Melons should be eaten alone. Fruit is best eaten alone.

2. *Proteins and Starches*

Proteins and starches should not be eaten together if food is to be well assimilated. Each of these combines better with greens than with fruits. Proteins include seeds (uncooked or fermented), sprouted seeds, nuts, legumes. Starches include potatoes, corn, carrots and other sweet tubers, avocados. Refer to *Cosmic Reawakening* by Artimia Arian for a detailed explanation of food combining.

3. *General Guidelines*

On a raw food diet the food combining rules are tricky when foods are sprouted, as once sprouted it is often difficult to know if the food is a protein or a carbohydrate (a starch). So let your body be your guide—gas, indigestion or constipation are signs of poor food combining. Do not eat more than one concentrate food per meal. Concentrated foods include: avocados, nuts and seeds, Essene bread, all cooked food, sprouted legumes such as sprouted garbanzos or lentils. Essene bread can be combined with avocado, a seed cheese, or a garbanzo dip, but should be eaten with a large green leafy salad to aid digestion.

Resting for 15–30 minutes after a meal facilitates digestion tremendously.

Avoid eating and drinking simultaneously.

Vegetable juices are digested in 15–20 minutes. Most fruit is digested in 20–30 minutes. Bananas, all melons and dried fruit are exceptions—they are digested in 40–60 minutes. A raw food vegetable meal takes 2–3 hours to digest. Be sure not to eat fruit until the previous meal is properly digested.

The Power of the Mind

Thoughts are energy and energy creates and affects everything. Thoughts are things, which manifest physically. Every thought has a shape, form, and color.

The subconscious mind does not differentiate between a thought and an actual event. The body reacts to a negative (or positive) thought as though it was actually experiencing the event.

Everything that we think is manifested externally in our bodies and in our lives. We are responsible for our own life and death and no virus or circumstance can bring illness upon us.

Anxiety and stressful thinking and living weaken the whole body, regardless of how pure and nutritional the diet.

Strong, pure, creative, happy thoughts build a strong, pure, balanced body. The body is a highly sensitive, finely tuned instrument, which responds to all thoughts all the time. Thought patterns (positive or negative) are producing positive or negative effects on the body constantly.

The body can be restructured and rejuvenated by changing one's diet and restructuring one's thought patterns. A different body plan has to be sent to the subconscious mind.

We are creators of our lives, not victims. Co-incidence, good or bad luck does not exist. Perfect order and justice exist in the universe. There is a just reason for everything.

Hatha Yoga, Pranayama and Meditation are great, powerful tools which enable one to purify and restructure one's mind. To master life one has to master one's mind. Mind mastery requires focusing only on positive, elevating divine thoughts.

Joy, freedom, love, knowledge, real bliss are our birthrights. We have to learn how to stop limiting ourselves; how to beware of what thoughts we are harboring; how to regain our force.

Yoga and live food are two potent tools, which purify and strengthen the body, emotions, mind and spirit.

Recommended Reading

Recipes for Longer Life — Ann Wigmore

The Hippocrates Diet — Ann Wigmore

Sunfood Diet Success System — David Wolfe

Light Eating for Survival — Marcia Madhuri Acciardo

978-0-595-39862-1
0-595-39862-6

www.ingramcontent.com/pod-product-compliance
Lightning Source LLC
Chambersburg PA
CBHW021547290526
45785CB00004BA/1933